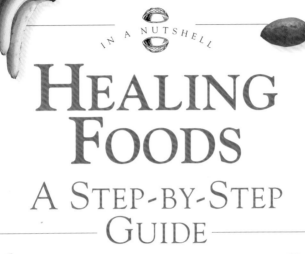

IN A NUTSHELL

HEALING
FOODS

A STEP-BY-STEP
GUIDE

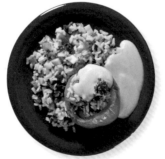

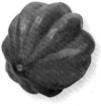

DENISE MORTIMORE

ELEMENT

SHAFTESBURY, DORSET • BOSTON, MASSACHUSETTS • MELBOURNE, VICTORIA

First published in
Great Britain in 1999 by
ELEMENT BOOKS LIMITED
Shaftesbury, Dorset SP7 8BP

Published in the USA in 1999 by
ELEMENT BOOKS INC
160 North Washington Street,
Boston MA 02114

Published in Australia in 1999 by
ELEMENT BOOKS LIMITED
and distributed by Penguin Australia Ltd
487 Maroondah Highway, Ringwood,
Victoria 3134

NOTE FROM THE PUBLISHER
Unless specified otherwise
All recipes serve four
All eggs are medium
All herbs are fresh
All spoon measurements are level

Designed and created with Element Books
by The Bridgewater Book Company Ltd.

ELEMENT BOOKS LIMITED
Managing Editor Miranda Spicer
Senior Commissioning Editor Caro N...
Editor Finny Fox-Davies
Group Production Director Clare Armstrong
Production Controller Claire Legg

THE BRIDGEWATER BOOK
COMPANY
Art Director Terry Jeavons
Design and page layout by Axis Design
Editor Jo Wells
Project Editor Caroline Earle
Photography David Jordan
Home Economy Judy Williams
Picture research Caroline Thomas

Printed and bound in Great Britain by
Butler and Tanner Ltd.

Library of Congress Cataloging in
Publication data available

ISBN 1 86204 381 7

The publishers wish to thank the following for
the use of pictures: Tony Stone Images
pp.6B, 10T, 34, 36BR, 47BR, 50BL.
The Image Bank pp.7T, 8BL, 14T.
CORBIS/Morton Beebe, S.F. p.32.

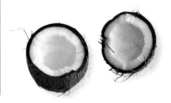

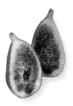

Contents

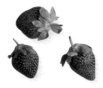

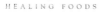
Introduction to optimum nutrition

RESEARCH HAS SHOWN *that the way to regain and maintain good health is through diet. The human body needs over 50 essential nutrients (vitamins, minerals, amino acids, fatty acids) each day, and by making the most of our diet, we can achieve youthful skin, clear thinking, and a strong, vibrant body. This book describes the "phytochemicals" that are found in fresh foods, and their individual uses in healing and disease prevention.*

ABOVE *Roasted vegetables with brown rice and watercress.*

Plants are dependent upon soil for their minerals and water supply. Today, the only way to be sure that food is wholesome is to eat organically-grown produce from an unpolluted, nutrient-dense soil. Although a totally organic diet may not be possible, the more organic food you eat, the more nutrients (and the fewer pesticides and pollutants) you will get, and the faster natural healing will occur. The phytochemicals found in fresh food are known to aid specific conditions. Antioxidants help with degenerative conditions, such as arthritis and heart disease, phytoestrogens ease

LEFT *Eating well will give you energy and vitality.*

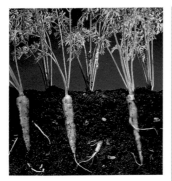

ABOVE **More organic
vegetables are now
being grown.**

The "phytochemicals" which
give food their color are
lycopene (red), betacarotene
(orange), curcumin (yellow),
chlorophyll (green), and
anthocyanidins (purple).

By incorporating a broad
"color mixture" of unprocessed
foods into your diet, you can
ensure that your body receives
the best raw materials to keep it
healthy. The suggested recipes
show how quick and easy it is
to achieve a healthy diet with
colorful and tasty combinations
of these vital foods.

female hormone problems, and a
whole range of substances have
been found to prevent cancer.

THE COLOR
CONNECTION
Research confirms
that many of the
attractive colors
in fresh foods are
related to a wide
range of health-
giving substances.

RIGHT **By
including foods
from the five main
color groups – red,
purple, green, orange,
and yellow – you will
guarantee a healthy
and attractive plate.**

Healthy eating

MANY OF US are hooked on the "fix" that carbohydrates and fats give us and fresh food is often an afterthought. But as your awareness of the positive power of good food grows, eating will not be only a pleasurable act, it will also become an event in which the body is given the vital nourishment it needs.

To ease the transition to a healthy diet, a slow start is suggested. Try a couple of the recipes in this book each week. The following plans give guidelines of what to aim for each day, each week and as a general eating plan.

BELOW *Fresh fruit makes a healthy snack.*

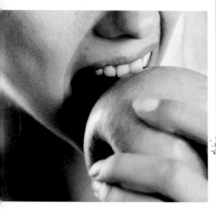

DAILY HEALTHY EATING PLAN

1 Five servings of fresh vegetables and fruit daily (vary them each day) and include one from each group: Brussels sprouts, broccoli, cabbage, cauliflower or kale: Carrots, peas, pumpkin, sweet potatoes, tomatoes, or watercress: Leek, garlic, or onions: Bilberries, black currants, black grapes or cranberries: Kiwi fruit, mangoes, papaya, peaches, or pineapples.

CABBAGE

MIXED SEEDS

2 A heaping tablespoon of mixed ground seeds and a little olive oil.

3 A small amount of mixed grains daily.

MIXED GRAINS

WEEKLY HEALTHY EATING PLAN

1 Oily fish three times a week, or three servings of ground flax seeds or oil for vegetarians and vegans.

2 A glass of soy milk or 2–3 ounces bean curd,

GLASS OF SOY MILK

three or four times a week.

3 Plain live soy, sheep's, goat's or cow's yogurt three or four times a week.

4 Brazil nuts and walnuts two or three times a week.

LIVE YOGURT

BRAZIL NUTS

GENERAL TIPS

SEAWEED

- Add sea vegetables to soups and stews and oat germ to cereals for extra minerals and vitamins.

- Gradually add beans, lentils, bean sprouts, pasta, whole grains, other vegetables and fruits, dairy foods (besides yogurt), white fish, eggs, and so on.

PASTA

- For maximum nutrient retention, only lightly cook vegetables and fruits or eat raw.

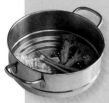

- Steam or stir-fry fibrous foods, such as string beans, to release nutrients.

- If frying is necessary, use olive oil or "steam-fry" with vegetable extract or stock or miso.

STEAMER

- Choose organic food or select foods close to their natural form.

- Keep processed food, confectionery, dairy food (except yogurt), and alcohol to a minimum.

- Avoid saturated fat, heated polyunsaturated oils, and excess sugar and salt.

OLIVE OIL

Green vegetables

GREEN VEGETABLES CONTAIN *chlorophyll, betacarotene, and flavonoids. Chlorophyll provides magnesium and vitamin K, both vital for healthy red blood cells. Betacarotene is an antioxidant, which helps the immune system, helps prevent cancers, and aids performance in cognitive tests. Flavonoids are vital for healthy blood vessels.*

Parsley, spinach, watercress, salad vegetables, and beet greens are rich in chlorophyll, carotenes, and flavonoids, as well as being good sources of calcium, iron, and vitamin C. Parsley, a traditional diuretic, can reduce the cancer-causing risk of fried foods. Green bell peppers, rich in vitamin C, contain substances which reduce the risks of heart attacks and strokes.

ABOVE *Asparagus is low in calories.*

Asparagus is rich in protein, vitamins B2 and C, folic acid, and potassium. It is a sedative and a useful diuretic, and is used to treat stress, indigestion, arthritis, and rheumatism.

Artichokes are low in calories and contain a starch called inulin which aids blood-sugar balance, and active ingredients that improve bile flow and protect the liver.

CAUTION

● Bell peppers, chili peppers, eggplants, tomatoes, and potatoes may aggravate arthritic symptoms in some people.

● For people with thyroid problems, "goitrogens" in brassicas interfere with iodine absorption. These are inactivated by cooking.

The skin of cucumbers contains silica, which is good for skeletal tissues and also for the complexion.

Dandelion greens increase the nutrient content of a salad, and are rich in betacarotene. The roots contain compounds that aid liver function, promote weight loss, support diuretic activity, and cleanse the blood. Dandelion coffee is made from the roasted roots.

BRASSICAS

Broccoli, Brussels sprouts, cabbage, kale, cauliflower, kohlrabi, mustard greens, collard greens, rutabagas, turnips, horseradish, and mustard

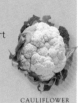

HEALTH TIP

Raw cauliflower flowerets eaten with a live-yogurt garlic dip can help to relieve indigestion, flatulence and constipation.

CAULIFLOWER

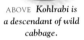

ABOVE **Kohlrabi is a descendant of wild cabbage.**

and cress have good levels of betacarotene, flavonoids, vitamins C, E, and K, calcium, iron, magnesium, boron, potassium, fiber, and chlorophyll. Eating cabbage three times a week can reduce your risk of colon cancer by 60 per cent. Broccoli and Brussels sprouts are particularly active against breast cancer. Brassicas contain glutathione and other phytochemicals which increase liver detoxification and can destroy harmful bacteria, such as Salmonella. Cabbage and cabbage water are excellent for soothing the digestive lining and stimulating the liver.

HEALTH BENEFITS

● Reduced risk of heart disease, stroke, high blood pressure, cataracts, anemia, spina bifida, cancers, and osteoporosis

● Helping detoxify the liver and improve bile flow

● Helping symptoms of PMS and the menopause

● Cleansing of the blood and maintenance of blood vessels

● Soothing the digestive tract

BROCCOLI

Avocado Dressing with Salad and Rice

PRECISE QUANTITIES *of vegetables are not given for the suggested salads—choose the mixture that you prefer and use whatever balance you feel looks most appetizing.*

INGREDIENTS

FOR THE RICE

generous 1 cup short grain brown rice

1 teaspoon turmeric

2½ cups stock

FOR THE SALAD

a selection of:

broccoli flowerets

arugula

iceberg lettuce

asparagus tips, steamed

beet greens

OR

white and green cabbage, shredded watercress

flat leaf parsley

OR

cauliflower flowerets

baby spinach leaves

fresh cilantro leaves

corn salad

FOR THE DRESSING

2 large ripe avocados, peeled and pitted

1¼ cups sugar-free, organic soy milk or oat milk

2 teaspoons sesame seed paste

juice of 1 lemon

pinch of paprika

pinch of black pepper

Makes about 2½ cups

AVOCADO

COOK'S TIP

To make the stock, either use an organic stock cube or miso paste.

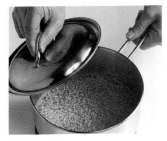

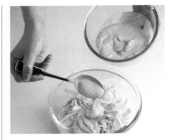

1 Rinse and drain the rice. Cook on a low heat in the stock and turmeric until the liquid is absorbed.

3 In a large bowl mix together the salad vegetables and spoon over a little dressing. Serve with the savory rice.

VARIATIONS

- Add a few freshly chopped Brazil nuts for extra flavor.

- Add potassium-based salt or tamari, if saltiness is required.

- Alfalfa sprouts, herbs, mixed bean sprouts, dandelion, and cucumber slices all combine well in these salads.

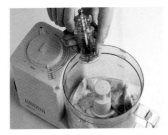

2 Mix all the dressing ingredients in a blender or food processor until smooth.

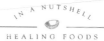
Carrots and carotene vegetables

THE ORANGE AND YELLOW PIGMENT *in vegetables, such as carrots, squash, red bell peppers, tomatoes, beet, and corn, comprises a group of phytochemicals called the carotenes.*

Carrots are a rich source of pro-vitamin A, including betacarotene. Two carrots a day provide more than enough betacarotene, plus vitamins C, E, some B vitamins and folic acid. They provide many minerals (calcium, phosphorous, sodium, iron, zinc, magnesium, potassium, and copper).

Raw carrots may inhibit Listeria, can reduce serum lipids and thus the risk of cardiovascular problems, and cut down the risk of lung cancer. Older, darker orange carrots

ABOVE *The colour of tomatoes and carrots is due to carotenes.*

contain more carotenoid antioxidants, which are fat soluble and more heat stable. Fibrous phytochemicals (lignans) help to balance estrogen activity.

SQUASH AND PUMPKINS

The dark varieties of squash, such as pumpkin, contain betacarotene, complex carbohydrates, and many of the B vitamins. They are also very low in calories with high levels

HEALTH TIP

Carrots are a good source of folic acid, which is essential during pregnancy.

CARROT

14

HEALTH BENEFITS

● Reduced risk of listeria infection, cardiovascular problems, heart disease, stroke, cataracts, cancer (lung and prostate especially)

● Rebalancing estrogen activity (PMS and menstrual problems)

● Provides nutrients important in pregnancy

● Boosting the immune system

● Helping gall bladder disease

● Treating and preventing constipation

● Improving night vision and preventing macular degeneration

of potassium and vitamin C. They protect against many cancers, particularly lung cancer

BEET
Beetroot has anti-cancer properties and contains calcium, iron, and vitamins A and C. It is an excellent blood cleanser. Beet fiber is good for bowel function and lowering cholesterol.

BEET

TOMATOES
Fully ripe tomatoes have high levels of betacarotene, plus vitamin C, potassium, and lycopene. A high intake of tomato-based foods has been linked to a reduction in risk of prostate and other cancers as well as a lower incidence of heart disease, stroke, and cataracts. The phytochemical coumarin in tomatoes, bell peppers, and carrots appears to prevent the formation of cancer-causing nitrosamines in the gut.

YELLOW VEGETABLES
Bell peppers and corn, as well as some spices—turmeric and mustard—contain curcumin, which protects against skin wrinkling and degenerative conditions, such as heart disease and cancer. Two further carotenes, zeaxanthin and lutein (found in corn, spinach, lettuce, parsley, and brassicas), can help reduce the risk of macular degeneration, a leading cause of blindness.

CORN

Spicy Vegetables and Beans

THIS DISH is rich in *betacarotene, protein, carbohydrate, and essential minerals, providing a balanced and nutritious meal.*

INGREDIENTS

3 tablespoons olive oil

1½ teaspoon fennel seeds

1 cinnamon stick

2 teaspoons chopped or dried oregano

4 garlic cloves, sliced

3 onions, cut into wedges

4 cloves

2 teaspoons ground cinnamon

1 teaspoon ground nutmeg

1 teaspoon black pepper

1 organic vegetable stock cube dissolved in ½ cup hot water

1 pound pumpkin, butternut squash, acorn squash or sweet potato, cut into chunks or slices

1 pound carrots, cut into long strips

2 fennel bulbs, cut into strips

1 pound mixed red kidney beans, lima beans, garbanzo beans (canned or freshly cooked)

½ teaspoon salt

4 tomatoes, peeled and chopped or 14 ounce can

1¼ cups vegetable juice or stock

Serves 4–6

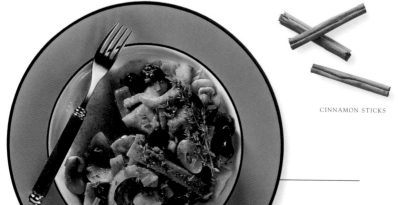

CINNAMON STICKS

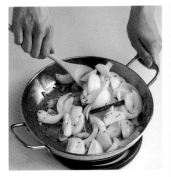

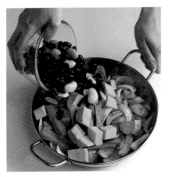

1 Heat the oil in a large heavy-based pan and add the fennel seeds, cinnamon stick, and oregano, then add the garlic and onion, and cook until soft.

3 Mix in the vegetables, beans, salt, and remaining juice or stock.

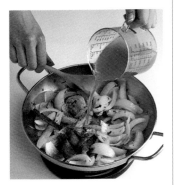

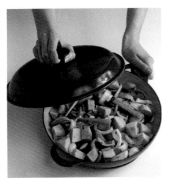

2 Add the cloves, ground cinnamon, nutmeg, pepper and ½ cup of the vegetable stock and fry for a few minutes.

4 Place in a large, covered dish and bake in a preheated oven at 350°F for about 40 minutes, or until the vegetables are tender. Remove and discard the cinnamon stick and serve, sprinkled with fresh herbs.

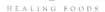
Phytoestrogen vegetables

FENNEL AND OTHER aniseed-flavored vegetables and spices contain chemical compounds which mimic the effect of natural estrogens. They boost low estrogen levels but at the same time reduce the overall effect of high estrogen levels. Phytoestrogens are important foods for both sexes.

Fennel is an excellent digestive aid. It is also a mild diuretic, probably because of its high potassium content. This quality also makes it a useful food for good kidney health and promoting weight loss. Fennel is effective in reducing high blood pressure and is also a useful source of folic acid for pregnancy.

COUMARIN

Fennel is higher in the phytochemical, coumarin, which helps to prevent cancer, than either celery or carrots.

LEFT *Fennel is a good diet food because a bulb contains only 50 calories per 3½ ounces.*

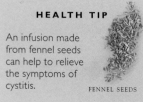

HEALTH TIP

An infusion made from fennel seeds can help to relieve the symptoms of cystitis.

FENNEL SEEDS

In addition to its anti-cancer properties, coumarin helps to tone the vascular system and enhances the activity of certain white blood cells.

HEALTH BENEFITS

- Rebalancing estrogen levels
- Helping symptoms of PMS, menstruation, and menopause
- Relieving symptoms of digestive complaints
- Cancer prevention
- Stimulating liver action

Diuretic vegetables

CELERY AND CELERY ROOT *are natural diuretics, helping the body to remove excess fluid.*

The high potassium content and diuretic effect of celery and celery root can help prevent and reduce high blood pressure. The increase in urine production eliminates excess uric acid and other unwanted substances common to joint complaints, such as gout. This diuretic effect may be why celery appears to reduce the onset and symptoms of migraine, although celery's stimulating effect on the liver may also help.

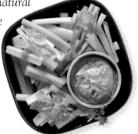

ABOVE **Celery served with a dip is a refreshing appetizer.**

HEALTH BENEFITS

- Preventing water retention and re-establishing mineral levels
- Reducing high blood pressure
- Helping symptoms of gout, joint pain, and migraine
- Preventing cardiovascular disease
- Kidney health
- Removing excess acid

The high levels of potassium and other mineral nutrients, such as sodium, make celery a great restorer of electrolyte balance in very hot weather or after a strenuous workout.

CELERY SEEDS

Celery seeds and their extract are useful for removing excess acidity from the body; this reduces joint pain and stiffness. Traditionally, the essential oil of celery and its seeds have been used for their calming effects, because they contain a natural tranquilizer. There is also some evidence that celery can help to combat cardiovascular disease.

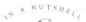

Fennel, Radicchio, and Feta Cheese Salad

THIS HIGHLY FLAVORED, *crunchy salad makes a refreshing treat for a summer lunch. Serve with warm crusty bread.*

INGREDIENTS

3 celery stalks, thinly-sliced

celery leaves

1 fennel bulb, thinly-sliced lengthwise

1 medium head radicchio, leaves torn

about 12 asparagus tips

½ cup small black olives

½ cup pimiento-stuffed green olives

1 cup diced feta cheese

FOR THE DRESSING

4 tablespoons extra virgin olive oil

1 tablespoons freshly squeezed lemon juice or lime juice

1 teaspoon fennel seeds, crushed

2 garlic cloves, very finely chopped

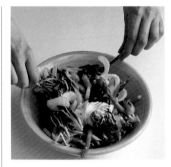

1 Combine all of the salad ingredients in a serving bowl.

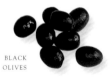

BLACK OLIVES

VARIATION

This salad is delicious with the garlic sauce on page 25.

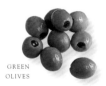

GREEN OLIVES

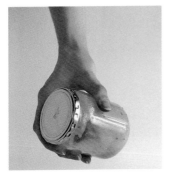

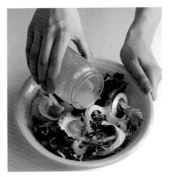

2 To make the dressing, shake all the ingredients together in a screw-top jar until thoroughly combined or whisk together in a bowl.

3 Pour the dressing over the salad and serve.

Garlic and the onion family

GARLIC IS THE WONDER FOOD of folklore; it contains around 200 biologically active compounds, many of which, such as antioxidants, are believed to be involved in the prevention of heart disease and cancer.

Garlic can significantly lower blood cholesterol (one raw clove a day can bring about a 9 per cent reduction) and prevent the formation of atherosclerosis. This and its ability to "thin" the blood lowers the risk of heart attacks and strokes and reduces blood pressure.

FIGHTING CANCER

Some Chinese studies indicate that eating large quantities of garlic can protect against stomach cancer; studies in America found that garlic was the most

GARLIC CLOVE

protective vegetable against colon cancer—even as few as two servings a week were effective.

The carcinogenic and poisonous effects of aflatoxins (made by molds), commonly found on poorly-stored peanuts, are also lessened by garlic. Its antifungal, antiviral and anti-bacterial qualities mostly relate to its high content of allicin.

One clove a day can be useful against coughs, colds, and sore throats and against toxic bacteria in the digestive system, in bladder infections, and overgrowth of the yeast candida. Its anthelmintic activity is useful for the treatment

GARLIC BULB

HEALTH TIP

Crush a clove of garlic with honey and lemon juice and add to a cup of boiling water as a home remedy for catarrh.

of intestinal worms, including threadworms in children. Its immune-stimulating effects have helped asthma sufferers and those with respiratory tract infections. Japanese research has even shown that memory and learning ability may be improved by eating garlic.

MINERALS

Garlic is very high in many of the trace minerals, especially sulfur, selenium, and germanium. Sulfur is an excellent liver detoxifier and blood cleanser.

Selenium is now considered to be borderline deficient in many individuals and is an important antioxidant, helping to boost liver function and eliminate harmful substances from the body. Its involvement in thyroid activity and blood-sugar control indicate that selenium, and probably other compounds in garlic, is very useful for those suffering from thyroid disorders and in diabetes.

Germanium is involved in metabolism and is able to improve energy levels, while reducing irritability and anxiety.

EATING GARLIC

Garlic is best eaten raw in salads, oven baked as whole cloves, or in sauces. If fried, it should be cooked without browning.

BELOW *Potato salad in garlic mayonnaise.*

ONIONS, SHALLOTS, CHIVES, AND LEEKS

These vegetables have many of the same properties as garlic, but to a lesser extent. Leeks are rich in fiber and have been used traditionally to treat sore throats and improve the voice. Onions, too, are extremely useful for respiratory complaints.

CLEANING LEEKS

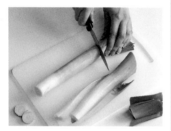

1 Remove the roots and any damaged green leaves.

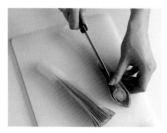

2 Slit from the top to the middle and rinse thoroughly.

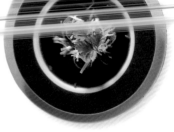

ABOVE *A traditional French onion soup.*

HEALTH BENEFITS

- Lowers cholesterol levels and high blood pressure

- Good blood cleanser

- Protects against atherosclerosis, heart disease, and stroke

- Balances blood-sugar levels

- Aids thyroid activity

- Helps eliminate heavy metals, such as lead

- Promotes detoxification

- Boosts the immune system

- Protects against cancer, especially of stomach and colon

- Kills bacteria, viruses, and molds/yeasts

- Kills intestinal worms

- Reduces irritability and the effects of stress/anxiety

Creamed Garlic Sauce

THIS SAUCE is versatile and delicious. *Serve it with salads, cooked vegetables, mixed cooked grains, pasta, baked potatoes, stuffed bell peppers, or stuffed tomatoes.*

INGREDIENTS

10 garlic cloves

1½ tablespoon olive oil

1 medium potato, finely chopped

generous 2 cups sugar-free, organic soy milk

2 tablespoons dark soy sauce

2 tablespoons Parmesan cheese

large pinch each of dried thyme, ground nutmeg and pepper, and ½ teaspoon salt

Makes about 2 cups

1 Peel the garlic cloves and soften by stir frying in 1½ tablespoon olive oil.

2 Combine all the ingredients, including the garlic and olive oil, in a saucepan. Cover and simmer for about 25 minutes, or until the potato and garlic break up when prodded.

3 Allow the mixture to cool, then process in a blender or food processor. Pour over the accompanying food of your choice.

Carbohydrate vegetables

IN GENERAL, starchy vegetables, *such as potatoes, sweet potatoes, and parsnips, are nature's tranquilizing foods. This property is related to the high carbohydrate content which has a soothing effect on the mind and emotions. However, too much carbohydrate, even from fresh vegetables, can cause imbalances in blood-sugar levels, which can lead to hunger and tiredness.*

To keep the balance right, starchy vegetables (as with pasta and other cereal products) are best eaten with fibrous vegetables and protein—a baked potato with baked beans, yogurt, or bean curd.

Very sugary, processed carbohydrates have a disastrous effect on blood-sugar balance, thus aggravating mood swings, irritability, and bad behavior. Excessive sugar intake

ABOVE **Curried parsnip soup is a warming dish.**

has been related to hyperactivity in children and aggressiveness in prison inmates. Potatoes, especially maincrop ones, have good levels of calcium, phosphorous, magnesium, iron, and vitamin C (mainly in the skins), with smaller amounts of zinc and the B complex of vitamins. Folic acid content is high, which makes them an excellent food for pregnant women and for children. The potassium content is exceptional, making potatoes very good for reducing high blood pressure and encouraging elimination of toxins by the kidneys. Their betacarotene

CAUTION

Never use potatoes that have green patches on them; this pigment is called solanin and it is a potential poison.

HEALTH TIP

Potatoes are very easy to digest and because of this are suitable for anyone with digestive problems, such as weaning infants and invalids.

content is reasonable, but much less than that of sweet potatoes.

Potatoes have a protein content similar to corn or rice, but also contain lysine, an amino acid often lacking in grains, which has been used effectively against cold sores. Potatoes can also benefit those suffering digestive problems, especially constipation and ulcers, chronic fatigue, and anemia.

SWEET POTATOES

Sweet potatoes generally have more nutrients than potatoes—good levels of magnesium, phosphorous, calcium, and iron, with moderate levels of vitamin C. Folic acid is high. The protein and potassium content are similar to potatoes, but betacarotene levels are far higher. The

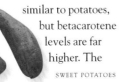

SWEET POTATOES

darker the orange pigment, the greater the antioxidant activity. Sweet potatoes are the richest low-fat source of vitamin E (good for cardiovascular health and clear skin).

PARSNIPS

Parsnips have very high levels of calcium, phosphorous, sodium, magnesium, and potassium. They have moderate levels of iron, zinc, and copper and some of the B vitamins.

PARSNIPS

HEALTH BENEFITS

- A natural tranquilizer
- Useful in pregnancy and for children
- Reducing high blood pressure
- Eliminating excess water
- Helping with digestive problems, constipation, and stomach ulcers
- Easing chronic fatigue (when well balanced with protein)
- Helping to build blood and prevent anemia
- Cancer prevention (especially sweet potatoes)
- Cardiovascular health
- Clear skin

Crunchy Oven Fries and Bean Curd Mayonnaise

THESE CRISPY vegetable wedges combine well with the mayonnaise to make a healthy and tasty snack or side dish.

INGREDIENTS

FOR THE FRIES

3 tablespoons olive oil

3 tablespoons tomato paste

1 teaspoon paprika

2 tablespoons miso paste

1 teaspoon pepper

2 large organic potatoes, scrubbed

4 large parsnips, scrubbed

sesame seeds

Serves 4–6

FOR THE MAYONNAISE

8 ounces fresh organic or silken tofu

1 tablespoon extra virgin olive oil

1½ teaspoons shoyu or tamari

½ teaspoon pepper

4 tablespoons lemon juice

3 tablespoons water

Makes about 1⅔ cups

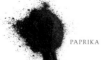

PAPRIKA

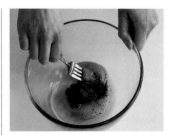

1 Mix the oil, tomato paste, paprika, miso paste, and pepper in a large bowl.

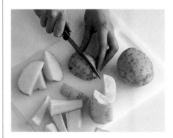

2 Slice the potatoes and parsnips in half lengthwise and then cut each potato half into six wedges, and each parsnip half into three.

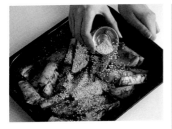

3 Toss the wedges in the oil mixture, making sure they are well coated. Place in an ovenproof dish and sprinkle generously with sesame seeds.

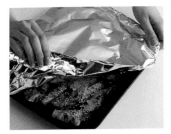

4 Cover and roast in a preheated oven at 400°F for 25 minutes. Remove the lid, return to the oven and leave the vegetables to brown for a further 10 minutes.

VARIATION

Use sweet potatoes instead of ordinary potatoes.

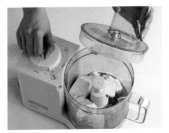

5 To make the mayonnaise, process all the ingredients in a blender or food processor until smooth.

Sea vegetables

MANY COUNTRIES, especially Japan, have harvested sea vegetables for thousands of years. Most edible seaweeds contain chlorophyll and more minerals than any other natural food. The growing conditions in the ocean depths provide rich deposits of nutrients and protect deep-sea plants from the harmful effects of manmade chemicals (although seaweeds gathered from the beach may contain pollutants).

Sea vegetables are fiber-rich and contain excellent levels of copper and iron for healthy blood, magnesium to assist in nerve and muscle function, calcium for healthy bones, potassium for the heart and fluid balance, zinc for a healthy immune system and reproductive health, iodine for active thyroid function, silicon for good skin, cobalt for formation of vitamin B12 and vitamins A, B complex (especially B12), C, and E. They are an excellent source of vegetarian protein and, at the same time, are low in calories. There are about 100 varieties of edible seaweed, of which the most common are listed below:

ARAME
Mild and rather sweet. Add to soups, stews, and stir-fries; good with bean curd.

ARAME

DULSE
This deep red seaweed has a strong, salty taste. It is popular in soups and salads, but it can be rather tough.

DULSE

HIJIKI

A strong, black variety. Crisp and tender, but may need longer cooking. Used in similar ways to arame.

HIJIKI

KOMBU

Brown and versatile. Can be used in clear soups, stews, stocks, and sauces and be pickled. Can also be dried, ground, and used as a condiment, thus adding many minerals.

KOMBU

pickle parcels, or with fish as in sushi. Also very good with bean curd. Rich in protein and minerals.

WAKAME

Available in strengths of flavor. Cooks very quickly, thus ideal for adding to soups, stews, beans, and other vegetables toward the end of the cooking time. Also good in salads. Can be ground and used as a condiment.

WAKAME

LAVER

An acquired taste. This seaweed grows just off the coast of south Wales and Ireland; a traditional breakfast dish of the Welsh. Also used to make laverbread.

LAVER

BELOW **When laver is simmered until it is a purée, it is known as laverbread.**

NORI

Available in "strengths" of flavor, it can be used in large "sheets" for making vegetable, rice, egg, or

NORI

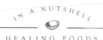
HEALTH BENEFITS

- Helping to reduce high blood cholesterol
- Balancing body fluids
- Protecting against arteriosclerosis
- Assisting thyroid disorders
- Has anticancer properties
- Contains anticoagulants for prevention of abnormal blood clotting
- Effective detoxifiers, especially for removing heavy metals from the body
- Low calorific content and good for weight loss
- Helping in cases of anemia, poor immune system, stomach ulcers, and treatment and prevention of osteoporosis
- Maintaining the healthy function of the nerves and muscles (including heart muscle)
- Keeping bones and connective tissue healthy
- Good for reproductive health

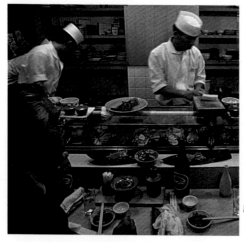

LEFT *Seaweed has long been part of the famously healthy Japanese diet.*

Brown Rice Cones

THESE MAKE an ideal starter *or can be served with salad, or steamed vegetables. They are particularly good with fish.*

INGREDIENTS

2 sheets nori seaweed, toasted

1⅓ cups cooked brown (or brown basmati) rice

½ bunch watercress, chopped

1⅓ cups grated fresh carrots

4 tablespoons sesame seeds, lightly toasted

1 tablespoon made mustard

1 tablespoon cider vinegar

1 tablespoon lemon juice

watercress, to garnish

Makes 8

1 Cut each nori sheet in half, and then cut each half into 4 triangles, giving 8 pieces altogether.

2 Mix all of the remaining ingredients together in a bowl.

3 Fold each piece of nori into a cone and use a drop of water to stick the overlapping corners to each other.

4 Fill each cone with the rice mixture and garnish with a sprig of watercress.

Cereal grains

GRAINS ARE the edible seeds of grasses—*wheat, rye, oats, barley, rice, millet, and corn. They are high in fiber, complex carbohydrate, polyunsaturated fatty acids, vitamins B and E, and many minerals (including calcium, iron, and magnesium). Most have high protein levels and many contain antioxidants.*

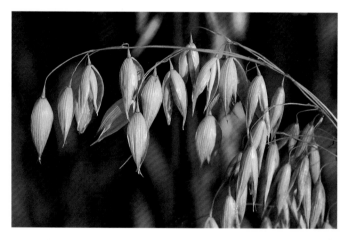

ABOVE **Oats contain**
lots of soluble fiber.

Wheat is a nutritious grain when used as a whole grain, burghul, and couscous, but wheat fiber eaten as "bran" or (too much) bread, can irritate the intestinal wall, impairing nutrient absorption. Intolerance to gluten is becoming common, but, fortunately, there are gluten-free grains—rice, millet, corn, tapioca, amaranth, buckwheat, and quinoa. Durum wheat, in pasta, is less allergenic.

Rye is very filling and is better tolerated than wheat. It has more fiber and less gluten; consequently rye bread is heavy and rises only slightly.

Oats are high in protein and have a soluble fiber—good for lowering cholesterol. Nutrients in oats stabilize blood-sugar levels, combat inflammation, and possibly prevent cancer. The polyunsaturated fatty acids in oatmeal help to ease inflammation and boost cardio-vascular, hormonal, and immune health.

OATS

Barley is rich in minerals and good for urinary infections, constipation, high cholesterol, cancer prevention, and also inflam-mation of the throat, esophagus, and digestive tract. Barley oil and rice oil contain powerful antioxidants for both healthy circulation and digestion.

BARLEY

Rice is high in protein and very nutritious. Wholegrain (brown) rice is the healthiest, and is useful,

WILD RICE

MILLET

particularly the short grain variety, for bowel detoxification. Wild rice contains more protein than oats or brown rice.

Millet is higher in protein than either wheat or rice and is alkali-producing. It is easily digested and rich in nutrients (especially silicon, which promotes healthy hair and skin). It also contains betacarotene.

ABOVE *Popcorn is made from the whole corn grain*

When popping corn and ground corn (used to make polenta and tortillas) are eaten, they provide the nutrients from the whole grain and are a particularly good source of zinc, essential fatty acids, and antioxidants.

Tapioca, arrowroot, sago, and amaranth are not true grains, but are easily digested foods ideal for convalescents. Quinoa is a perfect high-fiber, non-allergenic food. It contains twice the amount of protein found in rice and is rich in calcium, B vitamins, poly-unsaturated oils, and many other useful nutrients.

ABOVE *Quinoa can be used instead of rice to accompany savory dishes.*

Buckwheat (kasha) is high in protein, essential fatty acids, minerals, and vitamins. It contains rutin, a bioflavonoid, which can strengthen the walls of the capillaries and it is therefore useful to treat conditions such as chilblains and varicose veins. The antioxidants contained in buckwheat help to reduce high blood pressure and atherosclerosis. The lysine makes buckwheat complementary to other grains in providing high-quality protein.

BUCKWHEAT

HEALTH BENEFITS

● Treatment and prevention of constipation

● Energy boosting

● Reproductive and hormonal health

● Healthy blood

● Reduction of high cholesterol levels and high blood pressure

● Immune boosting

● Stabilization of blood-sugar levels

● Cancer prevention

● Keeping the urinary tract healthy

● Helping digestive problems

● Toxin elimination

● Prevention and treatment of osteoporosis

ABOVE *Cereals are a good source of energy.*

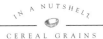
Quinoa Pudding

THE NUTRITIOUS and tasty *quinoa pudding is very easily digested and high in protein and fiber.*

INGREDIENTS

⅔ *cup quinoa,*
washed and drained

2½ *cups soy or almond milk*

2 *tablespoons manuka honey*

cinnamon stick

pinch of salt

2 *cups mixed strawberries,*
raspberries, mangoes and bananas

carton of soy cream

STRAWBERRIES

1 Boil some water in the base of a double saucepan.

2 Heat the milk and quinoa together over direct heat in the top section of the saucepan. When the mixture is just boiling, put the pan into the bottom section and reduce the heat to medium.

3 Add the honey, cinnamon stick, and salt. Stir well, cover, and simmer gently over low heat for 30–40 minutes, until the liquid is absorbed and the mixture is smooth and creamy.

4 Discard the cinnamon stick and pour into individual dishes. Serve with the fruit mixture and drizzle with soy cream if preferred.

Soy and other pulses

PEAS, BEANS, AND LENTILS *are staple foods for many vegetarians and vegans. All are high in carbohydrates and protein. The quality of protein in soy is actually equal to, and sometimes better than, animal proteins. Soy and beancurd are both good sources of phytoestrogens known to reduce the risk of hormone-related cancers, such as breast, ovarian, cervical, and prostatic cancer.*

An ideal intake for cancer prevention is around 1½ cups of soy milk or a good serving of bean curd four or more times a week. However, women who are pregnant, breastfeeding, or who suffer from endometriosis should not consume large amounts of soy products.

Soy products can reduce levels of harmful blood fats involved in heart disease, high blood pressure, and gall stones, and regulate bowel function and blood-sugar balance.

Bean curd is particularly rich in calcium, selenium, magnesium, and boron. Some research has shown a risk reduction of one-third for stomach cancer by eating a daily portion of miso soup. Traditionally, Japanese women use soy to strengthen their bones.

OTHER PULSES
Pulses include a wide range of beans, split peas, lentils, garbanzo beans, and peanuts.

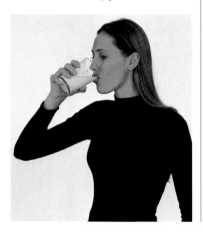

LEFT *Use soy milk as a low-fat, alternative to cow's milk.*

CAUTION

Soy beans can be allergenic in some people and may cause indigestion or headaches. Flatulence may occur when large amounts of beans are eaten—cook or use beans and peas with summer savory, fennel, or caraway seeds to prevent this.

HEALTH BENEFITS

- Lowers cholesterol levels and blood pressure
- Improves heart and circulatory disorders
- Cancer protection
- Blood-sugar balance
- Elimination of excess fluid
- Prevention of gall stones
- Helping symptoms of PMS and the menopause
- Prevention and treatment of osteoporosis
- Blood building and prevention of anemia
- Immune boosting
- Pregnancy and healthy reproductive organs
- Prevents constipation
- Relieves stress and tension

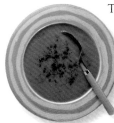

ABOVE **Split peas make a thick and nourishing soup.**

They can be used in soups, stews, burgers, "meat" balls, salads, for sprouting, or as vegetables. Beans eaten in their pod and raw are high in fiber and carbohydrate. Beans, in particular, are rich in potassium and very low in sodium and therefore have a mild diuretic effect. Their high levels of iron, chromium, molybdenum, and zinc are good for anemia and boosting the immune system. Beans and lentils are rich in folic acid—good for women planning pregnancy. Calcium, phosphorous, magnesium, zinc, copper, betacarotene, and vitamin C are also found in many pulses.

SPROUTED BEANS

Uncooked sprouted beans contain chlorophyll and carotenes, as well as many natural enzymes, RED LENTILS to help digestion.

Bean Curd Salad with Peanut Dressing

THIS CRISP AND CRUNCHY SALAD *in a coconut and peanut dressing is delicious with bok choy or another oriental vegetable, but Swiss chard is a good alternative.*

INGREDIENTS

3 medium-sized potatoes,
boiled until just "done" and cubed

1⅔ cups green beans,
halved and briefly steamed

13 ounces firm bean curd,
cut into 1-inch cubes

2 small heads bok choy, chopped

½ cup bean sprouts

1 small green cucumber, chopped

HOT PEANUT DRESSING

1 tablespoon olive oil

1 small onion, finely chopped

1½ teaspoons curry powder

½ teaspoon ground cumin

1½ teaspoons sweet chili sauce

2 teaspoons all-purpose flour

4 tablespoons crunchy peanut butter

scant ¾ cup vegetable stock

1⅔ cups can coconut milk

1 tablespoon brown sugar

½ cup freshly-shelled
peanuts, chopped

BEAN CURD SALAD WITH PEANUT DRESSING

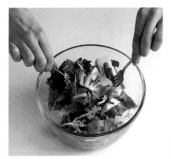

1 Combine all the salad ingredients in a bowl.

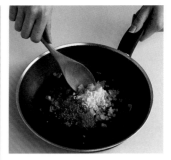

3 Add the curry powder, cumin, chili sauce, and flour and stir-fry for a further 2 minutes.

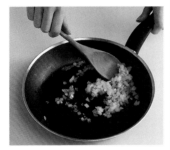

2 To make the dressing, heat the oil in pan, add the onion, and stir-fry until soft.

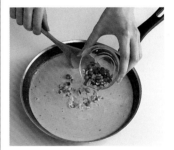

4 Add the remaining ingredients and heat, stirring constantly, until the mixture boils and thickens slightly. Drizzle over the salad and serve.

GREEN BEANS

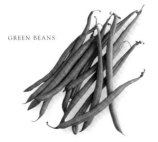

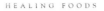
Seeds and nuts

NUTS AND SEEDS *are high in protein, carbohydrate, fiber, and polyunsaturated fats, with a whole range of minerals and vitamins. They are very rich sources of essential fatty acids and vitamin E.*

Nuts and seed oils are often used for salad dressings, but only the best quality should be used. Always store them correctly and use unheated. The most stable cooking oil is olive oil; which contains monounsaturates and vitamin E, vital for cholesterol balance and cardiovascular health.

MIXED NUTS

Sunflower, sesame, pumpkin, and flax (edible linseed) are the most nutritionally complete seeds. The first two are high in the omega 6 series of essential fatty acids; the latter two in the omega 3 series (found otherwise in oily fish).

HEALTH TIP

Whole flax seeds swallowed with water are a remedy for constipation.

LINSEED OIL

This oil has the best balance of essential fatty acids and is an excellent source of phytoestrogens.

The micronutrients in linseeds and other seeds include calcium, phosphorous, iron, copper, magnesium, potassium, zinc, and betacarotene; all contain some of the B vitamins.

Seeds are best eaten complete in salads and cooked vegetable dishes, lightly toasted or sprouted. Fenugreek seeds have an insulin-like effect and have been used to treat mature-onset diabetes.

SEED CHEESE

Crushed seeds make excellent "seed cheeses" (mixed with garlic and herbs) and "butters" (sesame paste).

PUMPKIN SEEDS

COCONUT

The coconut, actually a fruit, contains fat in a form instantly burned rather than stored. It has many nutrients and exceptionally high levels of folic acid. Eat coconuts fresh or as spreads, milk, butter, or cream. Coconut oil is high in vitamin E and phytoestrogens. Another true fruit with a nutrient profile more like a nut is the avocado.

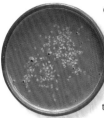

ABOVE *Sesame seed paste is the traditional sauce for felafel.*

NUTS

Nuts are best eaten freshly shelled, lightly roasted or as "creams," "nut butters," or dips. Walnuts have good amounts of essential fatty acids; others, such as Brazil nuts, are rich in selenium. Cashews are rich in copper. Almonds and hazelnuts contain calcium, magnesium, potassium, iron, zinc, copper, boron, E and B vitamins. Hazelnuts, cashews, and chestnuts contain betacarotene; Brazils, chestnuts, fresh coconut, and hazelnuts contain vitamin C.

HEALTH BENEFITS

- Lowering high cholesterol
- Helping to prevent heart disease and signs of aging
- Preventing constipation
- Helping with hormonal, nervous, and immune functions
- Healthy circulation
- Improving bone health
- Helping with thyroid activity
- Maintaining electrolyte levels
- Healthy skin and hair
- Relief from symptoms of PMS and the menopause
- Cancer protection
- Prostate problems
- Anti-inflammatory
- Preventing kidney stones
- Blood building and prevention of anemia
- Healthy muscle and nerve function

RIGHT
Sesame oil dressing with a crunchy walnut salad.

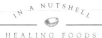
Savory Pumpkin Seed Pudding

THIS LIGHT AND GOLDEN *batter pudding is nutritious, tasty, and wonderfully filling when served with a rich gravy.*

INGREDIENTS

2 tablespoons olive oil

generous 1 cup pumpkin seeds

1¼ cups all-purpose whole wheat flour

2 large eggs

2½ cups soy milk

1 heaping teaspoon dried mixed herbs.

½ teaspoon salt

pepper

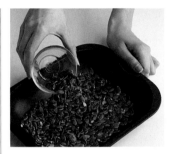

1 Put the oil and seeds into a shallow roasting pan and cook in a preheated, moderately hot oven, at about 350°F, for about 10 minutes, until beginning to sizzle and "pop" (not brown!).

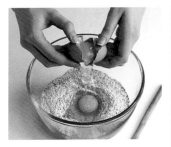

2 Process all the other ingredients for 30 seconds in a blender or food processor. Alternatively, put the dry ingredients into a large bowl and add the eggs.

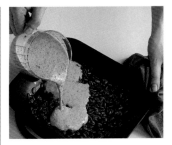

4 Pour this mixture over the hot seeds and bake for about 25 minutes, until risen and golden. Turn upside down and serve with a green vegetable, such as broccoli, and a rich gravy.

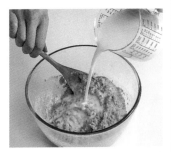

3 Gradually beat in the milk with a wooden spoon.

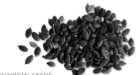

PUMPKIN SEEDS

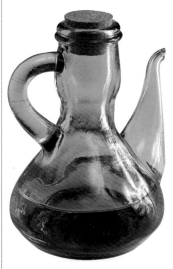

OLIVE OIL

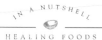
High-protein foods

MOST OF THE dietary protein *for vegetarians and vegans comes from cereals, pulses (especially soy), seeds, and nuts. Further protein may include dairy produce, eggs,* and *sometimes fish; vegans, however, refrain from using animal products.*

Heavy reliance on dairy foods may cause food intolerance, joint pain, heart disease, and a worsening of asthma, eczema, psoriasis, and catarrhal conditions. Try to minimize consumption of dairy products and use organic goat's and sheep's milk in preference to cow's milk products. Soy milk, soy cheese, soy cream, almond milk, and rice milk are all better alternatives.

CAUTION

Hard cheeses such as Parmesan are high in salt and lactose, and contain 30 per cent more saturated fat than softer goat's and sheep's cheeses.

EGGS

Eggs are a first-class protein. Although they are high in cholesterol, the yolk also contains lecithin which helps to metabolize cholesterol. In addition, eggs provide vitamins B, D and E, some zinc and reasonable amounts of selenium, iodine and iron.

LEFT *By drinking orange juice with a breakfast of eggs you will maximize iron uptake.*

Little iron is absorbed unless vitamin C foods or drinks are taken at the same meal.

YOGURT

LIVE YOGURT

Live yogurt is a high-protein food; vegans can use live soy yogurt instead.

Even those who are intolerant to cow's milk may find that they can eat cow's yogurt because the lactose (milk sugar) has been converted to lactic acid and the milk proteins made more digestible by the bacterial activity.

Live yogurt contains calcium, iodine, and a variety of health-giving bacteria, which improve the absorption of many minerals, help to maintain bowel health, and also reduce the absorption of microbial toxins and excess cholesterol.

Research has indicated that healthy intestinal bacteria can produce enzymes which are absorbed directly through the gut wall and work to enhance the body's immune activities.

HEALTH BENEFITS

LIVE YOGURT

● Protecting against harmful bacteria and their toxins

● Reducing the levels of yeasts, especially candida

● Reducing vulnerability to gastroenteritis

● Speeding up recovery from diarrhea

● Helping prevent urinary tract infections

● Helping prevent osteoporosis

● Restoring healthy gut flora after antibiotics

● Stimulation of immune function

● Helping to heal peptic ulcers

● Improving the levels of B vitamins, especially B12

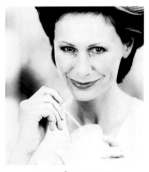

ABOVE *Live yogurt is easy to digest.*

OILY FISH

For the vegetarians who include fish in their diet and non-vegetarians, oily fish are a good source of protein. Mackerel, salmon, sardines, pilchards, kippers, fresh tuna, and herrings are high in omega 3 oils, which improve brain function.(Non-fish eating vegetarians and vegans can eat pumpkin seeds, flax seeds, and their oils for the omega 3 oils.) Along with some shellfish, they contain much iodine, selenium, zinc, and vitamins D and E.

For added calcium, consume the soft bones of canned fish. Canned or packet peppered fish have many of these oils.

BELOW *Fresh or smoked, mackerel is a delicious source of the vital omega 3 oils.*

HEALTH BENEFITS

OILY FISH

● Lower the risk of heart disease

● Reduce the risk of stroke

● Reduce high blood pressure and high cholesterol levels

● Reduce tendency to form blood clots

● Help remove the pain and stiffness of arthritis

● Help ulcerative colitis

● Relieve inflammatory skin conditions

● Reduce breast pain

● Prevention of some PMS and menopausal symptoms

● Help reduce risk of cancer

● Help improve brain and memory functions

Peppered Mackerel and Zucchini

SUCCULENT SMOKED MACKEREL *is combined with bell pepper, tomatoes, and zucchini in a white wine sauce. Brown rice, millet, and pasta all make excellent accompaniments to this dish.*

INGREDIENTS

1 tablespoon olive oil

2 garlic cloves, crushed

1 large onion, finely chopped

1¼ cups dry white wine

4 large pieces of smoked
peppered mackerel

1 red bell pepper, seeded and sliced

4 large tomatoes, peeled and chopped

1¼ cups sliced zucchini

1 tablespoon chopped parsley, to garnish

1 Heat the oil in a pan. Add the garlic and onion and cook until soft, but not brown.

2 Add the wine, bring to a boil, and reduce by half.

3 Flake the fish into bite-size pieces and mix with the bell pepper, tomatoes, and zucchini. Add to the pan. Cook until the zucchini are just tender.

4 Serve with rice and garnish with the parsley.

ZUCCHINI SLICES

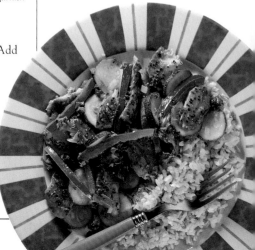

Berries, grapes, and cherries

BERRIES AND OTHER FRUIT *with a blue or red color are rich in vitamin C and the phytochemicals anthocyanidins, bioflavonoids, and proanthocyanidins, particularly the skins. They appear to inhibit the body's production of inflammatory metabolites—rather like aspirin, but without the gastrointestinal side effects.*

Strawberries and raspberries contain some effective phytonutrients, although strawberries have much more vitamin C, and provide coumarins and chlorogenic acid, which eliminate cancer-causing substances. Eating strawberries helps to cleanse the digestive system and also appears to help

HEALTH TIP

Plums and prunes are often eaten for their laxative effects.

whiten teeth. In addition, their boron content is important for hormonal and bone health.

Blueberries are good for the pancreas. Blackberries are a good source of iron and fiber, and contain some folic acid and vitamin E. Cherries are excellent at stabilizing blood-sugar levels, and are high in the minerals copper and potassium.

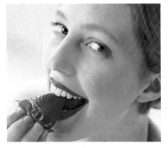

ABOVE **A summer treat packed with phytonutrients.**

GRAPES

They are effective against gout and are believed to help maintain skeletal tissues and skin to prevent premature aging.

Strawberries, grapes, raspberries, and cherries contain ellagic acid, which appears to block enzyme activity involved in cancer formation. Some American studies put strawberries at the top of a list of foods most closely linked to lower rates of cancer death among large groups of elderly people.

Cranberry juice contains hippuric acid, which aids recovery from urinary tract infections, prevents kidney stones and can help prostate problems. Blueberries, too, seem to have this effect. Substances in blueberries can prevent painful periods and protect the retina of the eye and the arteries against free radical damage.

Plums are a good source of carotenes, flavonoids, potassium, and iron. Black currants are rich in carotenes, fiber, iron, vitamin C, and potassium; they are excellent for helping to treat food poisoning and urinary tract infections, as well as being a traditional diuretic.

RED WINE

HEALTH BENEFITS

- Cancer prevention
- Help urinary tract infections, prostate and kidney problems
- Help cardiovascular problems
- Good for connective tissue and bone health
- Eye health
- Immune boosting
- Reduce free radical damage in arteries, capillaries, and joints
- Healing muscle damage
- Help psoriasis, arthritis, and other degenerative diseases
- Treatment of painful periods
- Soothing the digestive tract
- Inhibit food-poisoning bacteria
- Treatment of varicose veins and hemorrhoids

WINE

Red wine and red grape juice are especially rich in anthocyanidins and polyphenols, which reduce lipid oxidation in the blood and may offer protection against heart attacks.

Summer Dessert
with Coconut Cream

THE INTENSE COLORS *of the soft fruits used in this recipe make*
it an attractive dinner party dessert.

INGREDIENTS

4⅓ cups fresh blackberries, black grapes,
black currants, blueberries,
cranberries, pitted cherries,
strawberries, raspberries,
mixed fruit juice

Serves 4–6

COCONUT CREAM
1 ounce creamed coconut,
dissolved in 4 tablespoons hot water
1¼ cups soy or almond milk
1 tablespoon manuka honey

Makes about 1⅔ cups

RASPBERRIES

HEALTH TIP

Pollen
(in unfiltered
honey and
honeycomb)
may have a
desensitizing
effect on
hayfever or
asthma sufferers.

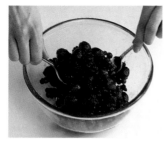

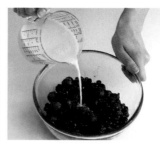

1 Mix the fruits together in a large serving bowl and pour on some fruit juice to add a little moisture.

3 Pour over the fruit and serve immediately.

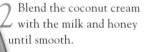

2 Blend the coconut cream with the milk and honey until smooth.

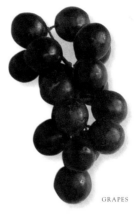

GRAPES

HONEY

Cold-pressed honey has many healing and antibiotic properties. Manuka honey, from New Zealand, can remove some bacteria, including the one thought to cause peptic and duodenal ulcers and, possibly, prevent stomach cancer.

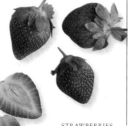

STRAWBERRIES

Tropical fruits

THE YELLOW PIGMENT *occurring in many of these fruits relates to the carotene content; the darker the color, the more betacarotene present. Tropical fruits are very rich in vitamin C and many of them* contain effective protein-digesting enzymes. Many also have antibiotic and anti-inflammatory properties.

Pineapples contain several compounds with marked antibiotic and anti-inflammatory effects. As a result, they are good for sore throats, fevers, and digestive problems. Pineapples also contain the protein-digesting enzyme bromelain, which is similar in action to papain in pawpaws.

These fruits are good for general soft tissue injuries, prevention of angina and high cholesterol, arthritis, indigestion, upper respiratory tract infections, and also trauma.

Substances in pineapple discourage the formation of dangerous blood clots, are anti-inflammatory, and possibly remove plaque from artery walls.

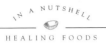

BANANAS

BANANAS

Bananas are full of nutrients, especially carbohydrate, potassium, vitamin B6, and folic acid. They are good for treating diarrhea, stomach ulcers, ME, exhaustion, and glandular fever, raised cholesterol, and prolonging energy for sports people. Bananas contain the amino acid tryptophan, which encourages restful sleep by boosting serotonin production in the brain.

PINEAPPLE

GUAVAS

Guavas are extremely rich in vitamin C, also B3 (nicotinic acid), phosphorous, and calcium and contain plenty of soluble fiber. Some of their uses include treatment for constipation, boosting immunity, heart and cancer protection, and reducing high cholesterol levels.

GUAVA

MANGOES

Mangoes are rich in vitamin C, betacarotene, vitamin E, fiber, potassium, iron, and B3 (nicotinic acid). They are excellent for maintaining a healthy skin, strengthening the immune system, and cancer protection.

KIWI FRUIT

Kiwi fruits have twice as much vitamin C as oranges and more fiber than apples. They are very rich in potassium and folic acid and

KIWI FRUIT

contain many natural enzymes. Kiwis are useful in the treatment of constipation, high blood pressure, depression, fatigue, poor digestion, and immune deficiency.

FIGS

Figs are rich in iron, calcium, potassium, copper, magnesium, manganese, betacarotene, and fiber and are effective against anemia, constipation, digestive problems, and cancer.

FIGS

PEACHES AND NECTARINES

Peaches and nectarines have high levels of vitamin C, potassium, carotenes, and flavonoids. They are easy to digest and can be used as a gentle laxative. The mineral boron is found in these fruits, which makes them helpful for hormonal and bone health. Apricots are rich in iron, potassium, and magnesium.

PEACH

Tropical Fruit Crumble with Vanilla Cream

CHOOSE YOUR FAVORITE FRUITS for this exotic hot dessert.

Add more fruit sugar to the crumble if you have a sweet tooth.

INGREDIENTS

1 pound 10 ounces selection
of fresh tropical fruit

fruit juice

fresh coconut, flaked

1 banana, sliced

½ cup brown rice flakes

scant 1 cup rolled oats

⅔ cup millet flakes

1 ounce wheat germ or oat germ

½ cup mixed chopped seeds
and nuts

2 tablespoons fruit sugar

Serves 4–6

VANILLA CREAM

4 ounces silken tofu

5 tablespoons soy milk

1½ teaspoons vanilla extract

1 teaspoon apple juice concentrate
or manuka honey

COCONUT

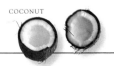

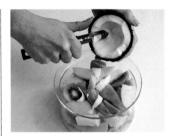

1 Wash and chop the fresh fruit. Place in an ovenproof dish and moisten with a little fruit juice.

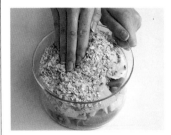

2 To make the crumble, mix all the dry ingredients together. Sprinkle over the fruit and press down lightly.

3 Bake at 375°F until the topping is just starting to brown.

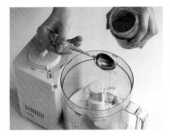

4 To make the vanilla cream, process the ingredients together in a blender or food processor until smooth.

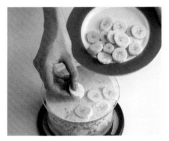

5 Pour the cream over the hot crumble and place the slices of fresh banana on top.

PAPAYA

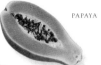

Food for common ailments

THE SYMPTOMS OF many common ailments can be greatly relieved by including certain foods in the diet.

Bad breath Parsley, dill, caraway seeds, aniseed

Colds and 'flu Dark green and carotene vegetables, shiitake mushrooms, fennel, celery, garlic, seaweed, oats, popcorn, beans, Brazil nuts, linseeds, pumpkin seeds, almonds, yogurt, strawberries, guavas, pineapples, mangoes, kiwi fruit

Constipation Carrots, green beans, beet, potatoes with skins, seaweed, barley, wholegrains, soy, pulses, whole linseeds, prunes, guavas, figs, kiwi fruit, peaches, nectarines, apricots, live yogurt

Coughs Fennel, garlic, onions, leeks, shiitake mushrooms, brassicas, pumpkin seeds, manuka honey, pineapples, mangoes, kiwi fruit

Cystitis Parsley, fennel, celery, barley, green beans, nuts, seeds, yogurt, cranberries, black currants

Fatigue Green and orange vegetables, potatoes, wholegrains, linseeds, bananas, kiwi fruit

Indigestion Asparagus, manuka honey, live yogurt, papaya

Insomnia Ripe bananas

Migraine Fennel, celery, garlic, berries

Skin problems Cucumber, turmeric, oily fish, corn, potatoes, sweet potatoes, millet, popcorn, soy, green beans, nuts, seeds, seaweed, bananas, guavas, pineapple, mango, cherries

Stress Asparagus, celery seeds, garlic, potatoes, oats, peas, nuts, seeds, berries, kiwi fruit

Upset stomach Brassicas, manuka honey, raw carrots, garlic, papaya, arrowroot, berries, pineapple, black currants

Water retention Asparagus, parsley, fennel, celery, potatoes, avocado, bananas, seaweed, pulses, black currants

Further reading

THE COMPLETE ILLUSTRATED GUIDE TO NUTRITIONAL HEALING, *Denise Mortimore* (Element Books, 1998)

HEALING FOODS FOR COMMON AILMENTS, *Dr Penny Stanway* (Gaia Books, 1995)

THE HEALING POWER OF FOODS, *Michael T. Murry*, ND (Prima Publishing, 1993)

NUTRITIONAL HEALING: A STEP BY STEP GUIDE, *Denise Mortimore* (Element Books, 1998)

THE NUTRITIONAL HEALTH BIBLE, *Linda Lazarides* (Thorsons, 1997)

THE OPTIMUM NUTRITION BIBLE, *Patrick Holford* (ION Press, 1997)

Useful addresses

The Vegetarian Society
Parkdale
Durham Rd
Altrincham
Cheshire WA14 4QG,
England

The Vegetarian Union of North America
PO Box 9710
Washington DC20016
USA

The Australian Vegetarian Society
PO Box 65
2021, Paddington
Australia

The Soil Association
86, Colston St
Bristol BS1 5BB
England

Farm Verified Organic
RR 1
Box 40A USA
Medina ND 58467
USA

National Association for Sustainable Agriculture
PO Box 768
AUS-Sterling
SA5152
Australia